IN PRAISE OF *GYMLESS FITNESS*

Gymless Fitness ('Yogalution') offers an effective methodology that builds on one's fitness step by step every day, all year round.

It removes the burden of time, travel and the cost of attending a gym.

The novel **DIY-back massage** is a master-stroke of genius.

The simplicity of this exercise programme assures consistent success.

Dr Sanjay Ganorkar
MBBS MS
Orthopaedic Surgeon and Yoga Practitioner
Nasik 422 001 India

My partner and I have positively benefited from Gymless Fitness beyond our expectations! We must say we are reaping the benefits in the most spectacular ways! Thank you again, Doctor!

Grace Jackaman, Cosmetologist
Belles & Beaus Semi-permanent MakeUp
West Sussex England (UK)

This is a fantastic exercise programme for people who are not gym-savvy and who prefer to workout at home.

Scientific and really well organised for the promotion of health and life longevity.

GYMLESS FITNESS

KEEP FIT, AT HOME, IN JUST 15 MINUTES A DAY!

DR SHREE VAIDYA
MD MRCP(UK)

Published by
Hybrid Global Publishing
301 E 57th Street
4th Floor
New York, NY 10022

Manufactured in the United States of America, or in the United Kingdom when distributed elsewhere.

Vaidya, Shree.
Gymless Fitness: Keep fit, at home, in just 15 minutes a day!
        ISBN: 978-1-957013-17-6
        eBook: 978-1-957013-18-3
        LCCN: 2022903472

Cover design by: Jonathan Pleska
Copyediting by: Dea Gunning
Interior design by: Suba Murugan
Author photo by: Spielman Photography

TheGymlessFitness.com

"Fitness isn't owned, it's leased. And rent is due every day." – Swamy Vigyananad

This book is dedicated to every able-bodied person, who is inspired to stay fit in all circumstances, to maintain their body machine in good working order by paying the lease fee of 1% of their day-time and a minimal effort.

The **Yogolution** model is dedicated to our times and to our lives, our busy lifestyle and all that comes with it, to 'here and now'!

Dr Shreedhar Vaidya
MB BS MRCP(UK) MD(Medicine)

CONTENTS

FOREWORD

I first met Doctor Shree at a virtual Zoom meeting during the peak of COVID-19 pandemic. He was able to raise the energy of the Zoom-room with his enthusiasm. I noticed his sharp intellect and innate ability to connect with the audience, capture their attention, and get them genuinely excited about his maverick ideas. So when Shree introduced me to his Gymless Fitness exercise plan, a simple but novel model for all ages and abilities, I immediately saw the practical application of this innovative, insightful work and how Doctor Shree simply enthuses others about fitness. His concept really resonates with the audience, particularly in these challenging times of lockdowns and ever-changing restrictions on our social mobility in the 'new normal'.

I have since come to know Doctor Shree Vaidya, MD, as a highly experienced physician from 'the land of YOGA' with polymathic interests, from anthropology-evolution, ecology, fitness, health, nutrition, vitality, wellness, longevity; to aesthetics and 1-hour puppet facelifts! Dr Shree is a result-oriented quick-learner and trouble-shooter with laser sharp focus.

As we all tread our paths on the journey of life, we are, on occasions, blessed by joining our steps along with those whose talent and intellect is exceeded only by their genuine desire to do good in the world by caring for the wellbeing of all. Doctor Shree is just such a person.

I am extremely impressed with Doctor Shree's self-explanatory 'Gymless Fitness' regime. It is not every day that a book comes along and inspires me. I've been publishing for quite some time now, so when Doctor Shree shared his idea, I knew it was going to light a million glows of fitness and vitality around the globe.

After reading this simple yet powerful book, I recommend it as a must follow! What makes this book so fascinating is that it offers a simple individually tailored process to keep you fit, indoors, and in just fifteen minutes a day! That's only 1% of your daily life! What an extraordinarily easy concept to break the natural inertia and time constraint in our busy lives!

Read this book and follow the simple dynamic activities in seamless succession. There is no way to do it wrong. The book contains a simple easy strategy to develop your fitness at your own pace, assisted by clear descriptions and helpful diagrams. You'll be so glad you started on this and the rewards will keep coming for the rest of your life!

I highly recommend Doctor Shree as the pioneering authority on 21st century evolved Yoga by Yogolution and Gymless Fitness.

Raymond Aaron, Physicist
New York Times Top 10 Bestselling Author

ACKNOWLEDGEMENTS

"GRATITUDE IS THE RENT WE PAY TO LIVE ON EARTH."

I would first like to thank my teachers who developed my analytical and improvisation skills, particularly **Dr. R. S. Wadia**, neurophysician, Pune and my post-graduate doctoral guide 1981-83.

I am deeply grateful to my late uncle, **Mr. Balwant Laxman Vaidya**, who pioneered teaching traditional yoga in India in the 1960's, and inculcated the habit of respecting and caring for the body through regular exercise.

I greatly appreciate my medical batch mates from 1975 MBBS batch in Pune, whom I acknowledge collectively; they have encouraged me to 'get this book out', have reviewed it and made suggestions and supported me all along. If I don't mention you individually, I include you personally. Thank you pals, this is for you.

I acknowledge leaders in the field of fitness, **Harvey Diamond** of 'Fit 4 Life', **Derrick Errol Evans** "Mr Motivator", **Fred Hahn** 'slowburn fitness', **Roger Sahouri**; and mentors & guides in the field of self-motivation: Tony **Robbins, Skip Archimedes, T. Harv Eker, Peter Sage** and so many members of the TLC – Transformational Leadership Council: **Jack**

Canfield, Martin Root, Dr John DeMartini, Mike Dooley, Cyndy Ertman, John Gray, Phyllis Haynes, Vishen Lakhiani, Sharon Lechtor, Mary Morrissey, Sheri Salata, Marie Smith, Carl Studna, Phil Town, Lynne Twist, JJ Virgin, Joe Vitale, David Wood, Sandra Yancey and Vahan Yepremyan, to name a few of the 100.

I am most grateful to the inimitable **Raymond Aaron**, who inspired, guided, and helped make my book a lot better; and to **Karyn Mullen**, who inspires Raymond.

I acknowledge help by writing & publishing coaches: **Chandler Bolt, Bennett R Coles, Jay Boyer, Jesse Krieger, Lea Constantine, Daniel Hall, Amy Collins, Joseph Michael** and **Sam Thomas Davies.**

Along the way, there have been many whom I would like to acknowledge for widening my horizons to the 'online' world: **Andrew Reynolds, Simon Coulson, Paul O'Mahony, Ross McKenzie, Adrian Morrison, Russell Brunson, Matt & John Rhodes, Ted McGrath, Mike Filsaime, Barry Plaskow,** and **William Souza.**

From the gratitude attitude, I fondly acknowledge leaders in all field of life, sports and politics who have moulded my mind-set in some way: form Socrates, Mustafa Kemal Ataturk, Lee Kuan Yew, Gandhi, Gorbachev, Mandela and PM of India **Narendra Modi.** I would like to admire here **Sunil Gavaskar, Kapil Dev, Sachin Tendulkar, Sir Vivian Richards, AB de Villiers, David Beckham, Lionel Messi, Cristiano Ronaldo, Rory McIlroy, Andy Murray**

---

and **Novak Djokovic.** I respectfully admire **Steve Jobs, Bill Gates, Jeff Bezos, Richard Branson, Elon Musk, Michael J Saylor, Donald Trump, Mukesh Ambani, HR Gaekwad** of BVG India, **Steven Fry** and **Dr. Clemen Chiang,** Ph. D, Founder & CEO of Spiking FinTech.

I think, these are the personalities I deeply want to acknowledge.

I take this opportunity to acknowledge in my first of many books, world thought and opinion leaders who have influenced my approach to fitness and life starting with **Oprah Winfrey, Joseph McClendon III, Amberly Lago, Scott Martin, Vani Hari** and of course, **Kim Kardashian.**

Finally, I acknowledge the contributors who helped me put together the book: the cover designer **Madhav** (Nepal), diagram illustrator **Subarna,** video editor **Sanjay,** text editor, formatter, graphic designer and all the back-office work-a-thoners under the auspices of **Karen Strauss** and **Sara Foley** of Hybrid Global Publishing.

Dr. Shreedhar Vaidya
MB BS MRCP(UK) MD(Medicine)

1

HOW AND WHY ALL THIS STARTED: LESS IS MORE!

"Necessity is mother of invention.
Laziness was the father!"

– Swamy Vigyananand

Congratulations for taking one significant step towards your own wellbeing, health and vitality through Gymless Fitness, the simplest, easiest, and modern method I have developed for you to stay flexible, fit, and active at any age.

So, take a moment to give yourself a pat on the back for taking action.

This book is somewhat unusual in that it is possible to start enjoying full benefits of the Gymless Fitness program by reading only up to chapter 2; simply by following instructions in the **Cheat Sheet** for Evol-Yoga! (You may skip to Chapter 2 now!) The rest of the book explains the concepts and movements in detail and makes the information complete, and the reader's experience wholesome.

The times we live in and the growing need to achieve more in less time-

- **The times we live in:**

Modern times are highlighted by fast life. Life, liberty, and pursuit of happiness has become so fast life, quick escape, and brisk pursuit of momentary happiness.

To be able to live and enjoy life to your fullest potential, you must be reasonably healthy, fit, and agile. The awareness of 'the need to invest time, energy, and money in the upkeep of our body's wellbeing, health, and vitality that enable you to enjoy a life of good quality and longevity has now well dawned upon us.

But increasingly, 'living life' comes in the way of 'enjoying life', what with the restrictions and 'the new normal' we all are facing due to the COVID-19 pandemic.

Today, the benefits of regular exercise towards improving one's health and maintaining wellbeing are as well-known as the injurious risks of smoking tobacco or drug-abuse.

The connection between regular exercise and health and fitness dawned on modern wise man Homo sapiens about the same time as the by-products of physically comfortable inactive sedentary lifestyle. This emerged with diseases of urban civilization, like obesity, osteoarthritis, stiffness, sprains and strains, chronic backache, frozen shoulder, diabetes, disabling stroke, and sudden deaths from acute heart attacks, or fatal coronaries, along with mental stress and depression.

Most urban people or desk-jobbers: people with a sedentary urban lifestyle, know that they must make time to do regular exercise in a structured manner. Some people have a jogging routine: in early morning, after work, or almost any time of the day and night.   Many have jogging-pals,-like commuting acquaintances whom they often run into on the jogging paths.

More serious and committed individuals have personal fitness-trainers, who map out and oversee an elaborate fitness program, a regime by setting goals and to achieve specific targets. 'Personal Fitness' is a big multibillion dollar industry today.

However, research has shown that many gym-attendances show a regular tendency to decline as time goes by. Membership renewal rates keep falling. And there are the logistics of getting to the gym at a particular time on a particular day, so many times a week. A small percentage never set foot in the gym of which they have bought membership! The cumulative carbon footprint of personal fitness by attending a gym is quite impressive. Of course, this would not apply to those few privileged with the luxury of space and resources of a customized personal gym at their sumptuous residence.

Generally, if your success at your day-job does not depend upon peak physical fitness, more likely, gym-membership –and regular attendance– are not your top priorities in the medium and longer term. Then there is the rush of busy life, family and social life take over, making heavy demands on your time.

'There is just not enough time!' Eventually, procrastination and human nature kick in...

As a UK National Health Service hospital doctor, having worked over eighty-three hours per week, while raising a young family together with my dedicated wife, I have been through the whole loop and grind of time-pressure on modern busy life.

Having experienced first-hand that uncomfortable feeling at doing nothing special exercise-wise, or throwing good money on bad gym-membership/s, that too, at no fault of the gyms, their increasingly flexible membership Terms &Conditions, or the excellent personal trainers; the burden of guilt became heavier.

The stress of this want-to-but-can't-do situation is not fatal, but it's quite an unpleasant 'gnawing' feeling one should do without. It must have some negative overall effect on the quality of our life. But let's not go on about the travails of busy life, personal priorities, inefficient time management, and the 'importance of regular exercise to one's health and wellbeing, the wisdom and evidence behind which are unchallengeable.

My Eureka moment: Yoga from ancient to modern:

Ancient yoga was still postures for long periods and slow breathing. EvolYoga is all dynamic stretches flowing into one another.

Let me tell you something about me.

I am a fully trained medical physician internist with over forty years' experience. I have lived in Europe for nearly thirty years. I come from India and my family name translates as 'doctor' or 'one who knows the Vedas'. I am the 5th or 6th generation of Ayervedic physicians in my family, and the first trained in modern medicine. (Ayurveda means 'Life Science'). I happen to have a family background of Yoga teaching – my uncle the Late B.L. Vaidya pioneered 'teaching yoga exercise at public classes' in India in the 1960s. In addition to having trained in the scientific discipline of modern 'allopathic' medicine, I have developed keen interest in evolution, anthropology, fitness, vitality and wellbeing, as well as astronomy, history, and philosophy. I see all these as serendipitous but helpful coincidences; but rest assured, I am not trying to teach you yoga, or sell you any magic herbs. They are too smart for a simple bloke like me.

I must make a strange confession to you. I am lazy...a bit too lazy to be really ashamed of it! I just work hard to 'afford my laziness' by being quite efficient in everything I do, to compensate for leisure.

And about twenty years ago, I applied the very same tactic to this 'want-to-but-can't-do, no-time-for-gym' conundrum.

- **How much is 1% of your day?**

Technically, a 24-hour day has 1,440 minutes, so 14 minutes 24 seconds is 1%. Let's say "under 15 minutes". Isn't 1% a good trade-off 'lease fee' to keep fit?

As a semi-desk-jobber myself, I decided at the outset that this activity must not take up too much of my time. I think about fifteen minutes every day should be a sufficient period anybody would not mind investing, in the upkeep of one's body-machine in working condition: fit, flexible, energetic, and ultimately healthier for longer.

I started by doing something that would not involve any gym equipment or coaching supervision by a gym or personal fitness instructor. I wanted something that people could perform at their own home-space by following simple instructions.

Then I thought about human anatomy, the common muscle groups and joints afflicted by stiffness, strains and sprains, and correlated it to the history of man's evolution from a quadruped (that is, walking on all fours) to bi-ped (like we walk now). I considered 'evolutionary ortho-kineto-aesthetics' ("the beauty & harmony of muscle-body movement during evolution") with special attention to our transition from quadrupeds to bipeds.

So I ended up developing a set of movements of joints using those muscles that we used more as 'quadrupeds' ('Q+'), but we seldom use since standing on our hind-legs and since our couch-potato lifestyle of sedentary urbanisation. I also included some movements that only us 'bipeds' can do ('B+'), but the 'quadrupeds' won't be able to do.

I call this process of evolution of bringing traditional yoga into 21st century as 'Yogolution,' and my exercise system 'Evol-Yoga' aka Gymless Fitness.

The funny bit is, it doesn't matter at all… zilch, if you do not understand any of this, because I've taken care of it all, for all of us.

Gymless Fitness is a simple and brief "Do-It-Yourself" exercise routine. This aims to achieve the goal to attain and maintain one's health, fitness, and wellbeing by simple, practical means: with zero dependence on any exercise equipment, or on being at a specific gym-place at a particular time on a particular day …so many times a week.

Of course, **Gymless Fitness** would also work for dedicated gym enthusiasts as 'plan B', when they can't make it to the gym for some reason on occasions.

An exercise tailored for each and every one of you!

The winning features are its simplicity and practical application for real benefit to all. And like your reflection in a mirror, this programme is automatically personalized for each and every one of you! For all ages, weight, shape, size! 'How could that be?' you may ask. Because **Gymless Fitness** routine depends on no external equipment, but the subject is working with their own body, and moving against their own body weight!

Imperfection would work as well as perfection! Please remember that consistency, discipline, and regularity would always trump perfection in Yogolution.

I have been personally practising this exercise routine I have developed, every morning over the past twenty years, practically from the beginning of the new millennium. I have tweaked it through a relentless process of improvisation and perfection with only these things in mind: simplicity, ease, and practical application for real benefit to all ages, for all abilities, body-shapes & bodyweights.

In summary:
I, 'Mr Lazy', have 'Done It Myself' for the best part of past two decades.

I spend just 1% of my day (that is less than fifteen minutes) for Gymless Fitness,

looking after my body by performing simple, easy, movements that are universal but provide personalized 'Gymless Fitness' benefit.

I have never suffered from any aches or pains, twist or sprains, or needed pain-killers for the past forty years.

You may call it personally 'tried & tested' **DIY Gymless Fitness.**

Or a fitness cheat-sheet for busy or lazy people.

Or a everyman's guide to easy-lazy fitness.

And that would perhaps include most of us!

And now I am ready to tell you all about it.

Cutting to the chase, let's have a quick peep at the cheat sheet.

2

THE GYMLESS FITNESS IN 1 PAGE: CHEAT-SHEET!

"Go to bed a little bit smarter every day!"
— Warren Buffet, Billionaire Investor,
'The Sage of Omaha'

"Go to bed a little bit fitter every day!"
— Dr Shree

Utkrant / Evol-Yogolution Gymless Fitness activities routine: 'cheat sheet'

0 **Getting up** off the bed: Cat camel – stretch like a cat with arms in front, bum up.

• **Standing posture**

1. **Sky-scratch**: vertical stretches of arms to ceiling or sky x10-15 ('warm up')

2. **Selfie-commend**: patting opposite shoulder blades on pushing elbows up & back x2

3. Standard **sun-salutes**: step lowering to ground face down & rising up. x4-14

4. **Elbow thrusts**-by-side: thrusting backwards arms folded at elbows x5

5. Straight lateral arms **swings-by-twisting** the torso at the waist, alternatively x7

6. 'Cricket-bowling action' **forward arm rotations** with outstretched fingers crossing in front x20+

7. Spider-web spin: swinging interlocked hands by chest clockwise & anticlockwise x10

8. **Elephant** trunk & head shakes: shake interlocked hands palms forward up/down x 7

9. **Butterfly-thrusts**: arms akimbo with forward thrusts of elbows x50+

10. **Dragonfly-thrusts**: arms parallel to ground, folded at elbows with fists facing each other; horizontal forceful traction away & punching thrusts x50+

11. **Sky-mining / 'cheetah sprint'**: Facing skywards, arms thrust up, flat palms, let fall in half-arc in front, bending elbows & thrusting back until 'heel-pop' x30+

12. **3D-head rolls & shakes**: like spinning top, clockwise & anticlockwise x3-5, shoulders relaxed along 3 axes, 'yes', 'no' & 'the Indian head-shake' @ x5

• **'On all fours': Crawling on palms & knees:**

13. **3D-head shakes:** nods along 3 axes, just as when standing, @ x5

14. **Sole claps:** alternate, @ x5

15. **Pony-kicks**: Bending knee up to chest & kicking forcefully as far back @ x5-10

16. **Push ups** (जोर) exhaling while going down by bending elbows till nose touches ground, then up in same swoop x 5-20 [may start with just one…]

- **Supine: on a firm flat surface, thin mat or a rug:**

17. draw circles & "figure-of-8" with toes of straight legs lifted from hips, anti/clockwise @ x 5-7

18. **Knee-diamond butterfly**: flapping movement of knees with soles joined,

19. **Bundled up**: then soles clasped in cupped hands, fingers interlocked: hold position for x3 deep slow breaths; then

20. **DIY-back massage**: in above posture, roll side-by-side until knees-to-floor x5-15

21. **Winding down**: x3 breaths: just RELAX! Imagine yourself as a feather, butterfly, sycamore seed twirling in the wind, recall & re-live the best moments from yesterday…

- **Standing up again ('getting ready for the day!')**

22. **Sit ups** (बैठका) holding opposite ear-lobules in index finger & thumb aka "super-brain-yoga" [in the US] x10-15, or w/backward arm swings [opp. #6]

23. **Backward arm-swings** [opposite direction of activity #6] x10-15

24. **SRT**: 'Sitting-rising test': Stand cross legged, pinch opp. ears. Now, sit down cross-legged & stand up without support. Super-advanced, if you can 'ground' your bum!

25. Finally, sit on a chair folding your arms & stand up on either foot, alternately.

Start small, by clock (15 minutes), or by ability /limit of physical endurance.

Breathe through nose, mouth closed, need not hold your breaths /grunt.

Ignore all skeletal noises so long as they are painless, [standard health-risk disclaimer]

Benefit is directly proportional to effort & duration, not dependent on speed or accuracy!

Enjoy healthy longevity while remaining fit.

Exercise is the 'rent you pay to your healthy body for living on earth'.

3

FREQUENTLY ASKED QUESTIONS

Why did the gym close down?
It didn't work out!
"Fitness has nothing to do with age"
— Virender Sehwag, Test cricketer

1. What is '**Gymless Fitness**'?
   Gymless Fitness is a simple, easy, convenient, short exercise program, without any need or dependence on visiting a Gymnasium facility.

2. Who is Gymless Fitness for?
   It is for anybody who would like to develop the good habit of getting exercise easily, simply, and without any recurring costs in time or other resources.

3. Is there any age limit for performing 'Gymless Fitness'?
   No. But it is recommended as "suitable for ages twelve onwards" for legal reasons.

4. Are there any height weight limits to 'Gymless Fitness'?
   No.

5. Are there any 'minimum ability' criteria for Gymless Fitness?
    Not really. Anybody able to sit, lie down flat, stand and walk without imbalance should be able to benefit from performing Gymless Fitness.

6. Do I need my doctor's permission to do this exercise?
    No. (See #21)

7. Where could I do this exercise?
    Anywhere. Indoors, by the side of your bed, in the lounge or outdoors on the lawn or by the swimming pool. In any space 2m wide by your height is enough.

8. Do I need a special dress or shoes?
    No. You may perform Gymless fitness in your pyjamas. We recommend a lower garment with thin elastic waistband. Belts and buckles are not advisable.

9. Is there any specific time of the day for Gymless Fitness?
    No. Ideally it is most beneficial in the morning on an empty stomach and on an empty bowel. But it could be performed at the office during lunch break, before eating any lunch!

10. I am very busy. Is Gymless Fitness for me?
    Yes. Gymless Fitness has been specifically designed for people on the go.

11. I am rather lazy. I don't 'fancy' exercise. What about me?

Perfect. Gymless Fitness is ideal for people averse to long tedious workouts.

12. How long does it take to perform 'Gymless Fitness'?

It takes under fifteen minutes. We all get 1,440 minutes in one day of our life. The program is designed to take up just about 1% of that time. (14 minutes 24 seconds to be precise. One may adjust the number of repetitions of each exercise to finish within fifteen minutes, just stop at fifteen minutes in whatever stage of the exercise, or carry on longer. It is totally flexible.

13. How can you claim that this exercise program is 'tailor-made to each individual of any age, or size'?

Because no external aid, weight or appliance is used, the person is just lifting or handling one's own weight, to the gram! It cannot get more personalized than that!

14. What are the advantages of Gymless Fitness to the users?

Gymless fitness achieves a reasonable quality of fitness, flexibility and stamina simply, conveniently, with minimum effort, and without any recurring costs of costume, Gym membership, and the logistics of transporting to and from the Gym.

15. Are there any other benefits?

Sure. Performing Gymless Fitness regularly would not only make one fit, but would mitigate or delay onset of common joint problems like frozen shoulder, cervical spondylosis, spinal kyphosis, scoliosis, hip-knee and ankle arthritis, back sprains, neck sprains, torticollis, and many other skeletal discomforts.

16. Anything else?
    One may not need separate time for 'meditation' if one were so inclined. There would be cumulative health, economical and eco-friendly benefits to mankind and the planet as a whole.

17. How much training is required to master 'Gymless Fitness' exercise?
    Very little.
    Gymless Fitness aka Evol-Yoga is the 'fast-food model' blend of traditional Yoga and aerobics workouts.
    - It is possible to start exercising just by reading and understanding the 1-page complimentary summary of the program, made available freely for benefits to mankind and the planet as a whole.
    - One could attain reasonable mastery by just reading the descriptive chapters in the book "Gymless Fitness".
    - Finally, it is possible to learn everything there is about "Gymless Fitness" by watching the three short videos within just ONE day!

18. What is Evol-Yoga (Utkrant Yoga) or Yogolution?
    Evol-Yoga is the concept of exercising those muscles, which humans have stopped using or under-using due to change in posture during

evolution from crawling-on-four to walking-on-two feet. ('Utkranti' is Sanskrit for 'Evolution')

19. There are several 'Yoga' programs available everywhere. What is so special about Gymless Fitness aka Evol-Yoga?

Ancient Indian Yoga places emphasis on postures, positions, and maintaining each of them for a few minutes (static), while Evol-Yoga is about dynamic movements and repetitions.

Also Evol-Yoga has been developed in the 21st century with conscious consideration to exercise those muscles & postures that humans have lost use of after changing from quadruped to biped posture only about 250,000 years ago. ('Evolutionary orthokinetics')

20. Is this 'calisthenics', then?

It matches Calisthenics ('Beautiful Strength') in principles, but in practice, Evol-Yoga differs from calisthenics in two aspects:

One, it does not involve jumping, running, climbing, balancing or gymnastics. Secondly most of the movements are different from traditional ancient calisthenics as performed in P.E. routines in schools or military training tests.

21. Are there any other specific restrictions for performing Gymless Fitness?

Gymless Fitness is not suitable for persons with history of miscarriages, in third trimester of pregnancy, with chronic persistent vertigo and imbalance, large hiatus hernia; or surgical or ballistic metal in their spine.

4

THE BEGINNING OF YOGOLUTION

"Health is the vital principle of bliss, and **exercise,** *of health"*

– James Thomson

"Health is the principle of vitality, and **fitness,** *of health"*

– Swamy Vigyananand

Anthropological Background of Evol-Yoga:

Ever heard of 'Nevolution'?

There is plausible evidence and understanding that our bodies developed over a long period of time to the present posture and abilities. **Evolution** is a concept by which every living organism adapts to its surroundings to be able to survive & breed successfully. They instinctively rely on subtle changes in their bodies that occur randomly, which we now know, by 'genetic mutations' (change). Obviously, those born with a change in physical appearance that is a beneficial 'improvement' for survival would naturally survive better (than those born without that mutation), and thus have the survival advantage and the best chance to breed and pass that genetic change to their next generation. Thus evolution is a continuous, extremely slow but continuous process of self-improvement in living beings.

A few hundred thousand years and generations ago, our human species experienced a break-out in this self-improvement, especially when we started to stand on our hind-legs, instead of crawling on all fours. Our hands-free tool-wielding worked wonders for our progress, also helped by the growth of the thinking and imagination parts of our brains; and development of language etc. Instead of adapting to our surroundings like all the other living beings, we started to control, change and adapt our surroundings to suit us! We became the masters of our environment. We built houses, farmed land, stitched clothing, and developed cuisines! The rest is, as they say, history! Man the wise had arrived.

Our mastery of our environment had many advantages in terms of our physical comfort, but counterbalancing disadvantages to our physical abilities. Our body suffered from our industrious progress, so did the environment and most other species on planet earth. (The rest of the universe doesn't seem to care...)

While me made strides of progress in general quality and standard of life enjoyment & leisure; the moment we started controlling our environment, our rapid progress –in the past 2,000-5,000 years– meant, from an evolution aspect, we overtook ourselves! The physical self-improvement of our body gotsort of arrested at the 'quadruped' stage, that is, when we were crawling on all fours– and from early biped stage, when we were, as cavemen, chasing game to hunt for our every next meal.

Artificial progress stopped our natural self-improvement! Due to the exponentially high speed of our progress in controlling our surroundings, we appear to have stopped evolving, we have been going backwards in terms of physical health and ability, stamina and vitality! Even our longevity appears to have peaked.

I call this turning point –when the speed of human progress overtook the slowness of evolution, or self-improvement in human biology– as 'nevolution'. Nevolution is 'relative evolutionary standstill'. Nevolution is a non-process: or non-progress, and non-improvement'.

How has 'nevolution' affected our bodies, fitness and well-being?

We get out natural health and fitness potential from our parents, whose genes we share. Quite impressively, human evolution has packed a lot of resilience, reserve, a lot of 'juice' or battery-life into our species! This would explain why some lucky people seem to get away with extreme indulgence, slothful living, smoking, and gluttony with little obvious damage to their body. But these are very rare exceptions, the rest of us get ravaged by environment and time!

Quite simply, the root of all our diseases of urbanization: obesity, osteoarthritis, diabetes, high blood-pressure due to rigid arteries, coronary heart disease due to narrowing and blocked arteries, leg cramps, chronic backache, frozen shoulder ...all are in this non-process of nevolution.

Because of our urbane lifestyle, we have stopped using some muscles to move the joints in our bodies for the purpose they had developed at the time of nevolution, we have been suffering from all the ailments, aches and pains and the general lethargy and unfitness by their disuse. Some of us consume too many calories, don't burn them off enough, smoke tobacco, and abuse alcohol, which all works against our physical health, fitness, wellbeing, and vitality.

5

THEORY AND CONCEPT

"A feeble body weakens the mind"
                                    – Jean-Jacques Rousseau

"A fit body strengthens the mind"
                                    – Swamy Vigyananad

What is fitness?

It is not just the absence of illness, or basic metabolic health, but also vitality, agility, alertness and the ability to 'flow'!*

(*The concept of 'flow' is credited to Mihaly Csíkszentmihályi in The Psychology of Optimal Experience, he outlines his theory that people are happiest when they are in a state of flow—a state of <u>concentration</u> or complete absorption with the activity at hand and the situation.

The "Flow +4% challenge" is the way to keep stretching your comfort-zone.)

Basics about Yoga as a practice of exercise:

'Yoga' means 'method' and 'yukti' is clever method: trick, or 'hack'. [Ancient Vedic' Yoga emphasises on postures of bodies called 'awastha', held for longer periods as 'aasana' and breathing regulation exercise called 'Pranayama' or 'life-breath-flow'. While Yoga has emphasis on static postures, often uncomfortable and strenuous, testing one's balance, etc.. Evolved Yoga or 'Evol-Yoga' is a dynamic concept that simply brings Yoga into the 21st century.

What is Evol-Yoga (Utkrant Yoga) or Yogolution?

Evol-Yoga is the concept of exercising those muscles, which humans have stopped using or been under-using due to change in posture during evolution, from crawling-on-four to walking-on-two feet. ('Utkranti' is Sanskrit for 'Evolution.') It also includes some movements that only we bipeds can do, but the quadrupeds won't be able to do.

You could also say that I have created a modern version of calisthenics and ushered traditional Indian Yoga-postures into dynamic 21st century by **Yogolution: DIY Gymless Fitness.**

Reflection on and of mother nature

Understandably, the movements reflect common activities in nature and draw their names from similar movements of various creatures in the wild:

- **Spider-web spin: If one approaches a spider perched at the centre of its web, at first the spider vibrates the whole web by rapid spinning in a circle and scurries away only if the threat persists, despite this show of power-spin.**

- Elephant trunk arms swings: exactly as the name suggests.

- Butterfly-swings: like the action of butterfly wings in flight.

- Dragonfly-thrusts: like the action of dragonfly wings in flight, a lot, lot slower...

- Cheetah sprint: Remember a cheetah's hunting sprint in any wildlife video. Imagine the movements (Q+) of the two forelimbs of the cheetah ...then rotate the picture 90° clockwise to upright... and 3-10 times slower! In effect, you are recreating that hunter's sprint-on-4, to your-activity-on-2 (B+), but in vertical direction, with some difference in the sequence of limbs, sequential for the cheetah and simultaneously in our exercise. Also our elbows go way back, the cheetah's need not.

- Pony-kicks: Just like a pony (or mule or zebra) kicking with its hind legs.

- Knee-diamond butterfly: similar to 'butterfly-swings' of legs.

So, let's get started! Let out the animal in you!

6

DETAILED DESCRIPTION OF EACH ACTIVITY: PART 1 (STANDING)

"Learn the most useful skill as if your body-house is on fire"

– Swamy Vigyananand

Consistency: "My fitness journey will be a lifelong journey."

– Khloe Kardasian

Detailed description of each activity: Part 1 (Standing)

The **Cheat Sheet** in Chapter Two gives a good overview of the program.

That would be sufficiently enough for some to get going.

Basics: You would need: Time, space, and you!

The best time I would recommend is after morning ablutions, a visit to the loo and before the bath or shower and breakfast. (Avoid within two hours of eating during the day.)

Remember to stretch and do a **cat camel** when you get out of bed.

All you need to begin with is a flat area the size of your body-print (arms raised height x arm stretched width) anywhere, bedroom, lounge, lawn, outdoors; A floor gym mat or firm thick-pile rug would help, especially if hard floors bother your knees or back.

Yes, fifteen minutes and a very minimal basic urge to live the longest, the healthiest, and the fittest life humanly possible, on the cheap!

If wearing clothes, simple, loose, pyjamas or leotard or shorts would be fine.

Music: If you prefer, listen to any music of your choice, soothing or energetic. Silence is golden.

Start small, by clock (fifteen minutes), or by ability: to your limit of physical endurance.

Try to cover all, or as many activities, even with less number of repetitions.

Benefit is guaranteed: directly proportional to effort, not dependent on time, or accuracy!

Enjoy healthy longevity while remaining fit.

CAT-CAMEL
माजर्रऊष्ट्रकम्

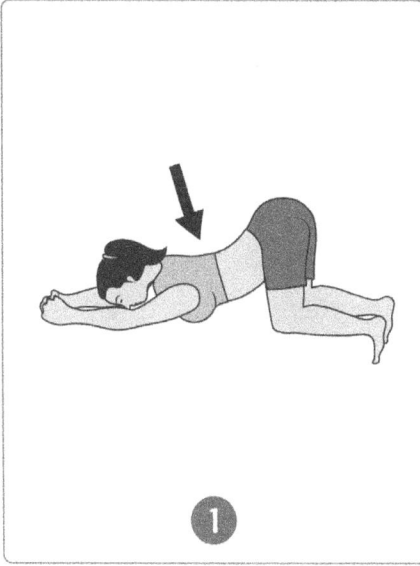

Always 'do & don'ts':

Keep it simple. Stretch slowly and lazily until you get in the swing of the repetitions.

Always breathe through your nose, mouth closed; no need to hold your breath or grunt.

You may ignore all skeletal noises so long as they are painless.

[usual disclaimer of liability]

Instructions for individual exercise:

1 **Sky-scratch**:   (warm up stretches)

   Body posture: standing,   feet   shoulder-width apart

   Head: facing forward, looking ahead

   Arms: by the side, neutral

   Palms: facing the body.

   Activity: Raise both arms above your head stretching reaching as high up as possible, with elbows straight. Revert to starting posture.

   Repetitions: 10 – 15

SKY-SCRATCH
ताडासन

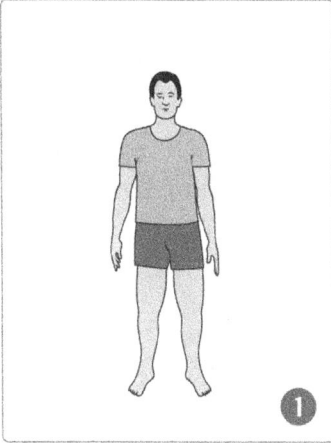

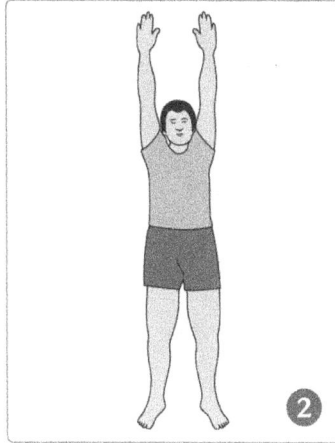

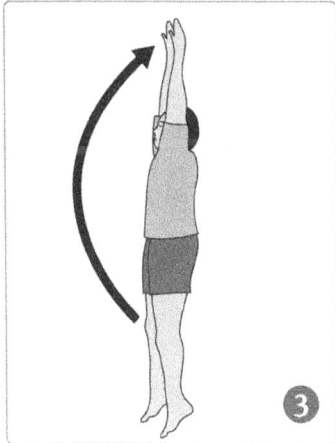

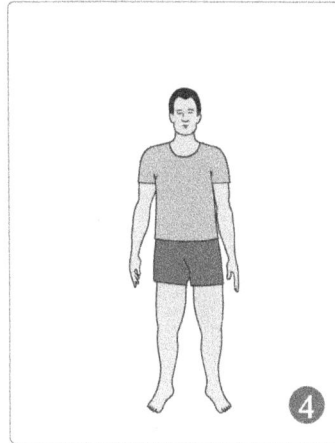

2 **Selfie-commend**: patting   opposite   shoulder
                   blades
   Body posture: standing, feet shoulder-width
                   apart
   Head: facing forward, looking ahead
   Arms: by the side, neutral
   Palms: facing the body.
   Activity: Raise each arm alternately above
                   your head
                   Fold at elbow to reach opposite
                   shoulder-blade
                   Pull the elbow backwards with
                   the other hand
                   Give 3-5 pats on your shoulder
                   blade
                   Revert to starting posture
   Repetitions: 2
   Tip: Start by cupping opposite
                   shoulders with your palms.

SELFIE-COMMEND
अपरस्कन्धस्पर्शम्

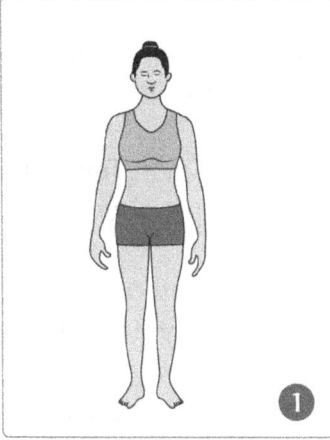

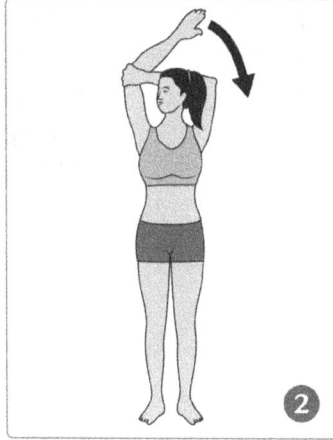

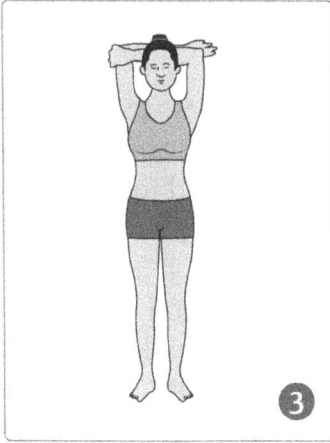

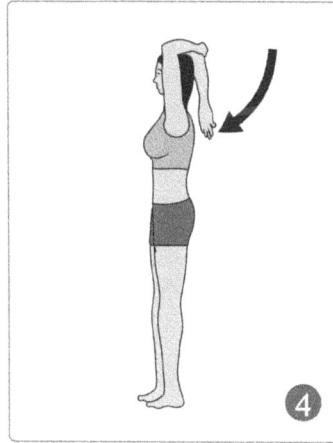

3 Standard	stepwise lowering to ground face
sun-salutes:	down & rising up.
Body	standing, feet shoulder-width
posture:	apart
Head:	facing forward, looking ahead
Arms:	hanging by the side, neutral,
Palms:	facing the body
Activity:	This is broken down in **Ten steps**:

1. Raise both arms above your head
2. Bend forward & stoop to touch the ground with your palms / fingertips
3. Stretch one leg behind as far as it goes, arching your back and head facing forward or upwards
4. Stretch the other leg by the side of first leg, resting whole body on just palms and toes
5. Arch backwards (Bhujangasana = cobra pose)
6. Gently touch and rest your forehead on the floor, trying to avoid chest or belly flopping to the floor as well. This is the salutation pose of 'Namaskaram'. Now we begin to reverse or undo this salute
7. Raise your head back to cobra pose (Bhujangasana) as in #5

SUN-SALUTES
सूर्यनमस्कार

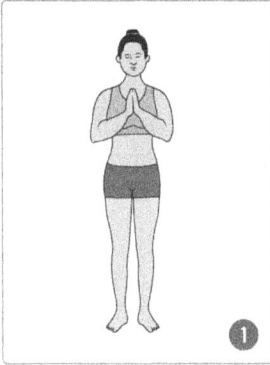

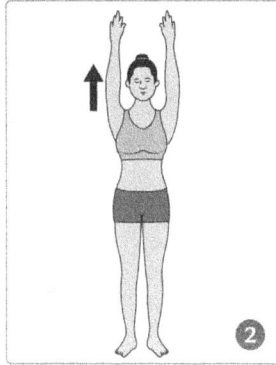

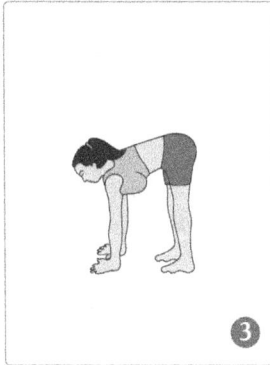

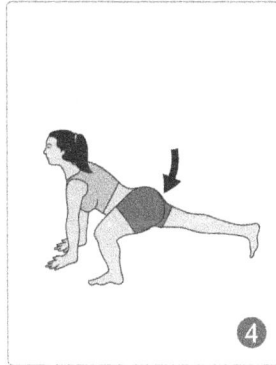

SUN-SALUTES - FROG POSE
सूर्यनमस्कार - मंडूकावस्था

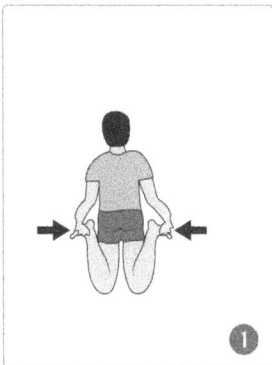

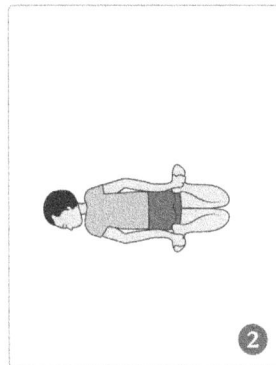

8. Bring forward one leg to original standing spot
9. Bring forward the other leg to get into stooping position at #2
10. Stand upright, arms by side as in the beginning. Revert to starting posture.

Repetitions: 4 – 12

Tips: You may alternate the legs at **#3, 4, 8 & 9.**

At **# 6** relax your arms by the side of the body and rest your whole body on the floor once, bend knees so you can grab your ankles and give a gentle stretch so that your heels touch the outsides of your thighs.

Hold positions **# 7, 8 & 9** for a second longer and give yourself a stretch in that position.

ONE-KNEE-BENT POSTURE
सूर्यनमस्कार - एकजानुवक्षप्रणिपात

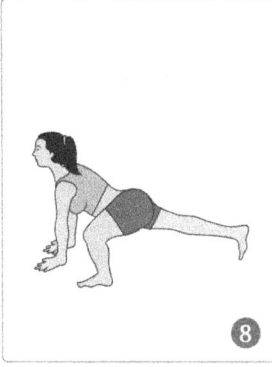

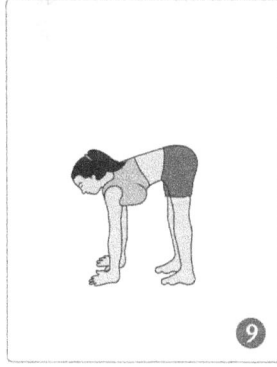

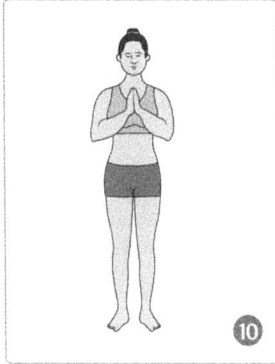

4 Elbow

thrusts-by-side:	thrusting folded elbows backwards
Body posture:	standing, feet shoulder-width apart
Head:	facing forward, looking ahead
Arms:	by the side, bent halfway at elbows, forearms horizontal
Palms:	rolled in fists
Activity:	With arms by your side and bent at elbows halfway, forearms horizontal, thrust your elbows backwards firmly as far as they would go. (If they meet behind your back, you are a flexible 'rubber-person'!)
	Revert to starting posture.
Repetitions:	5 – 10

ELBOW THRUSTS-BY-SIDE
अर्धगोमुखम्

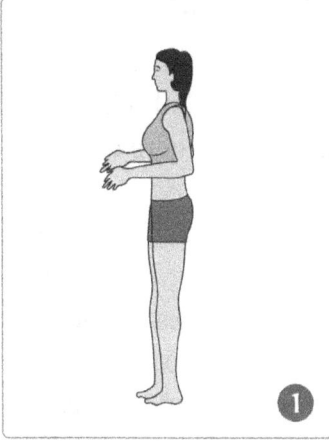
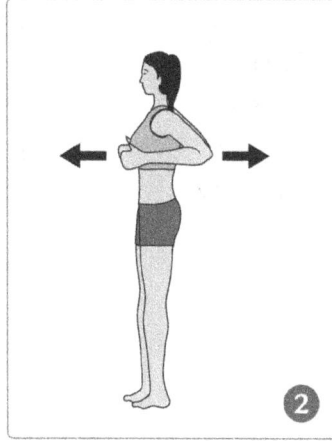

5 Straight arms **swings-by-twisting** the torso at the
   waist, alternatively

Body posture:	standing, feet wide apart for good balance
Head:	facing forward, looking ahead,
Arms:	by the side, loose flail relaxed,
Palms:	facing the body, fingers together.
Activity:	Twist at waist, alternately turning to either side with arms swinging and flinging freely, raised in near horizontal plane. You should be able to see just beyond midpoint behind your back and cover 'the whole circle' of your surroundings in the range of your vision.
Repetitions:	5 – 10
Tip:	Take extra care for a firm grip on the floor and maintain your balance.

STRAIGHT ARM-SWINGS-BY-TWIST
कटिचक्रम्

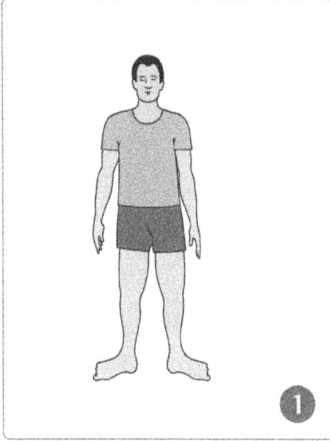

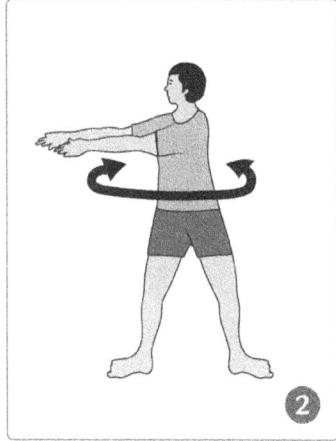

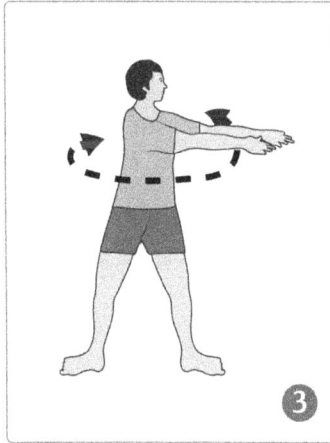

6 Cricket-bowling action **forward arm rotations:**

Body posture: standing,   feet   shoulder-width apart

Head: facing forward, looking ahead

Arms: by the side

Palms: facing the body, fingers stretched like fangs

Activity: Swing both arms backwards, bring overhead and down from the front (imitating the bowling action of a cricketer) to draw full circle in the air with your outstretched fingers

Repetitions: 15 – 30 continuous, non-stop.

Tip: You are doing it perfect when your fingers would touch, or better still, criss-cross like cogs in front of your face because of orientation of shoulder joints.

FORWARD ARM ROTATIONS
स्कंधचक्रम्

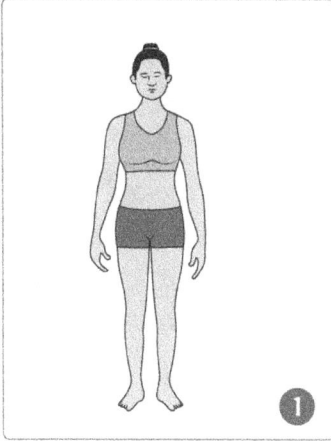

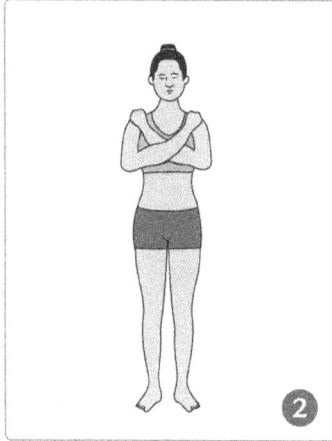

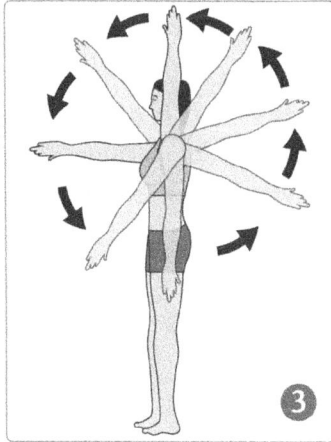

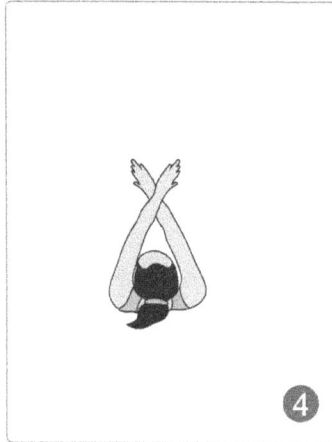

7 Spider-web spin:

Body posture: standing, feet shoulder-width apart

Head: facing forward, looking ahead

Arms: hanging, meeting in front

Palms: facing the body, fingers interlocked.

Activity: Swing the interlocked palms to draw full circle clockwise in front of your body, bending and straightening alternate elbow to keep arms close by your chest in frontal plane.

Revert to starting posture.

Repeat anticlockwise.

Repetitions: 10 each, continuous, non-stop.

Tip: During each rotation, your interlocked palms should be passing outside your shoulders.

SPIDER-WEB SPIN
तंतुनाभिका

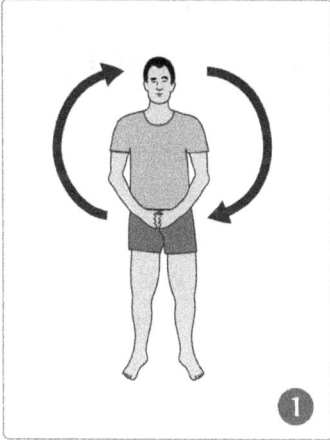

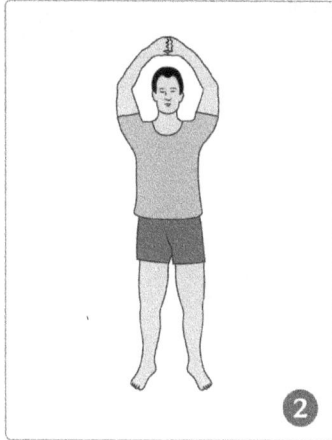

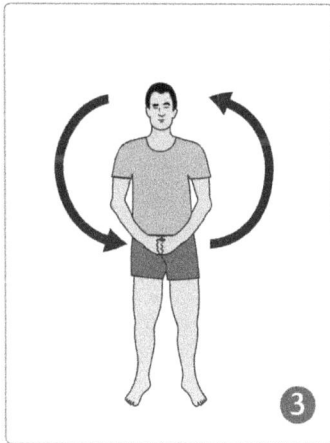

8 Elephant Trunk & Head Shakes:

Body posture:	standing, feet shoulder-width apart
Head:	facing forward, looking ahead
Arms:	in front, horizontal straight ahead, elbows straight
Hands:	with fingers interlocked,
Palms:	facing forward, away (thumbs pointing downwards.)
Activity:	move the interlocked arms up and down in an semi-circular arc, followed by moving head forward down & up with both arms outstretched as above.

ELEPHANT TRUNK & HEAD SHAKES
हस्तिशुंडाशिरान्दोलनम

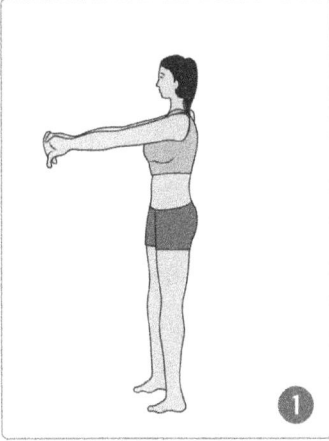

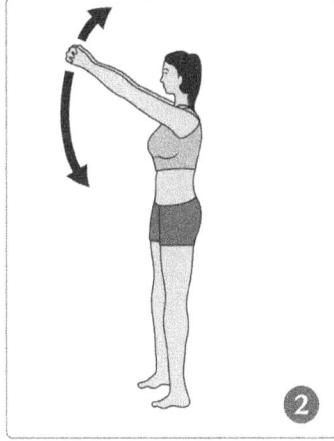

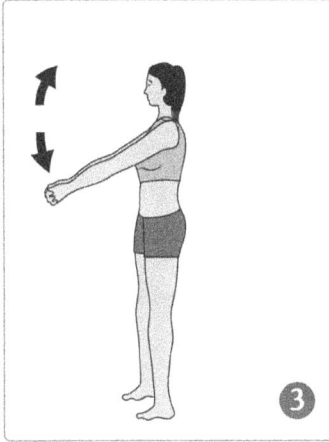

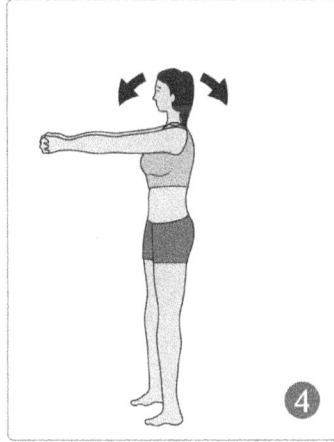

9 Butterfly-swings:

Body posture:	standing, feet shoulder-width apart
Head:	facing forward, looking ahead
Arms:	akimbo, hands on waist, elbows folded out like wings
Palms:	gripping the waist lightly, thumbs in the dimples of the sacro-iliac joints.
Activity:	Swing the elbows forwards and backwards in rapid flapping action without losing the grip on your waist.
Repetitions:	25 – 50 continuous, non-stop.

BUTTERFLY-THRUSTS
प्रजापति शलभिका

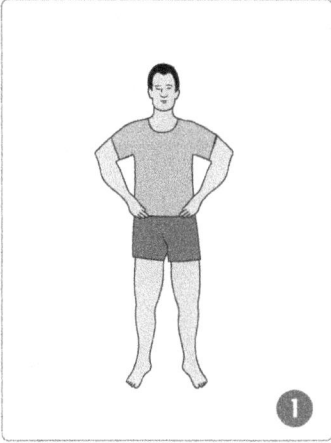

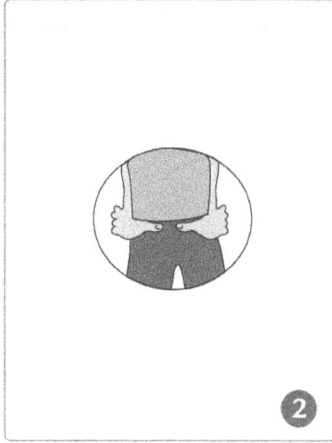

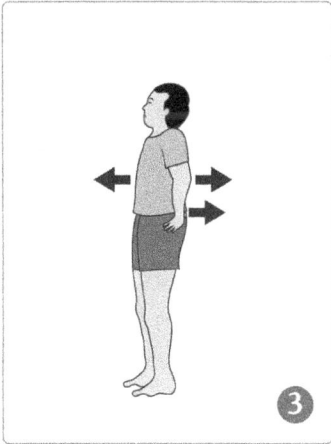

10 **Dragonfly-thrusts**:

Body posture:	standing, feet shoulder-width apart
Head:	facing forward, looking ahead
Arms:	raised to shoulder level parallel to ground, elbows fully folded
Palms:	made into light fists, almost meeting in front of your chin
Activity:	pull away the fists apart by stretching the elbows backwards, then pull forwards to starting position in punching thrusts & then forceful traction away, and so on
	The aim is to thrust the elbows as far back as possible, feeling the stretch in front where the ribs meet the breast-bone (sternum).
Repetitions:	25 – 50 continuous, non-stop
Tip:	Pay attention that the elbows are high horizontal and don't fall towards hips by relaxation of shoulders

DRAGONFLY-THRUSTS
व्याधपतंगकम्

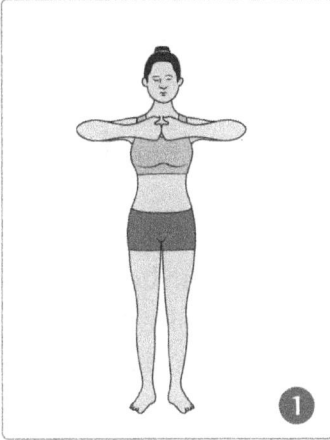

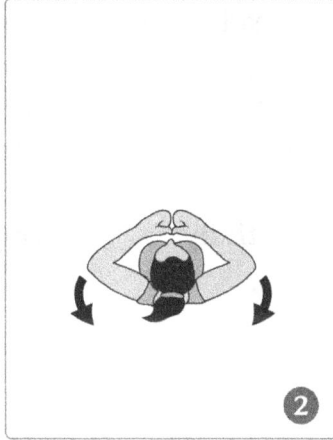

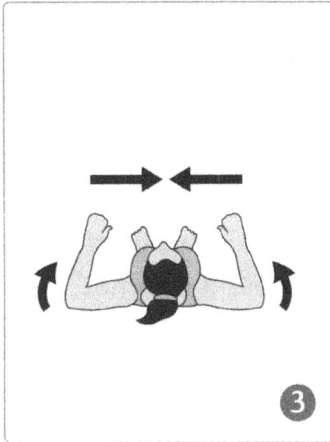

11 **Sky-mining / Cheetah sprint:**

Body posture:	standing, feet shoulder-width apart
Head:	facing forward, looking up to ceiling or sky
Arms:	by the side
Palms:	facing backwards, fingers closed like a paddle.
Activity:	Facing skywards, lift both arms by the side of your body, thrust them up into the sky, flat palms now facing forwards, then let them fall in front of you in half-arc, palms facing down until you revert to starting posture; but continuing the swing backwards, now bending elbows & thrusting as far back as they would go. The focus is on backward elbow-trust, the aim being to lift them as high as possible behind one's back at the end of the thrust, feeling the stretch in front of the shoulder, just where the bicep muscle begins.
Repetitions:	20 – 30 continuous, non-stop.
Tip:	Do not worry if at the beginning, your neck 'clicks' painlessly'. (It will stop clicking after you get into a routine…)
	Stop and skip if uncomfortable or hurting.

You would know you are doing this right, as your heels would momentarily get lifted off the floor by the momentum of your downward-&-backwards arm swing.

SKY-MINING 'CHEETAH SPRINT'
उपव्याघ्ररथम्

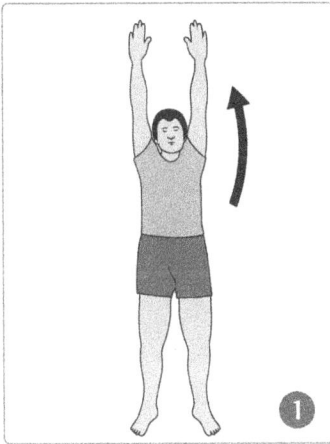

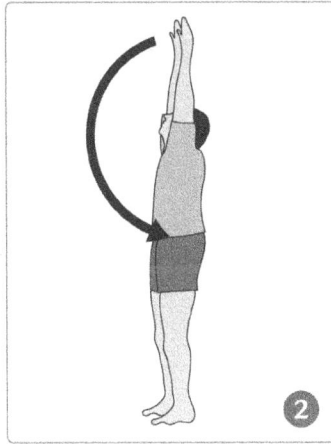

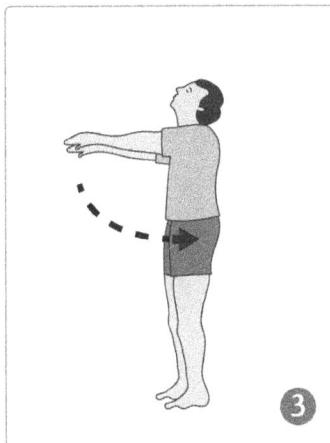

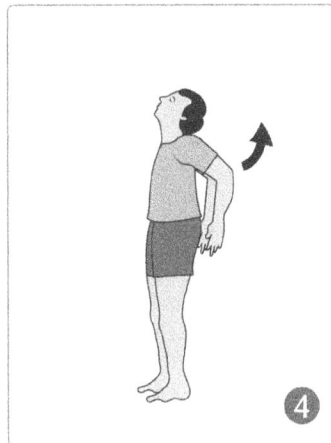

12 A: 3D Head rolls:

Body posture: standing, feet shoulder-width apart

Head: facing forward, looking ahead

Arms: behind the back,

Palms: facing backwards, fingers interlocked (as possible.)

Activity: Relax and roll your head pivoting on the neck 'like a spinning top', clockwise then repeat anticlockwise.

Repetitions: 3 – 5 continuous

Tip: Start slowly.

Ignore any sounds from neck so long as they are painless

Stop and skip if uncomfortable or hurting.

Your shoulders would tend to shrug up, but your arms interlocked behind your back would ensure they remain low and relaxed.

3D-HEAD ROLLS & SHAKES
शिरग्रीवासंचालनम्

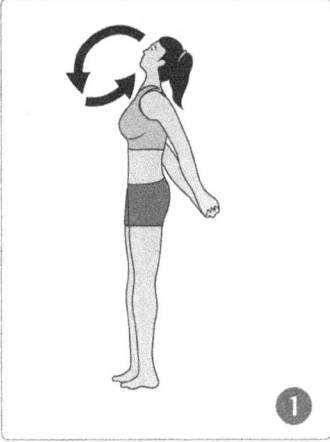

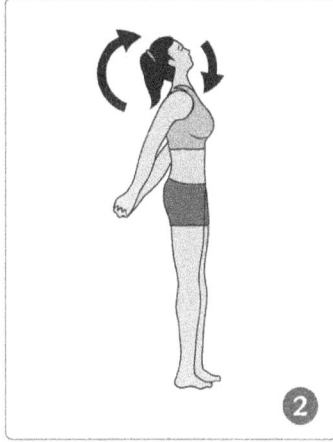

12 **B: 3D-head shakes:** [along 3 axes]

Body posture: standing, feet shoulder-width apart

Head: facing forward, looking ahead

Arms: behind the back,

Palms: facing backwards, fingers interlocked (as possible.)

Activity: Shake your head along 3 axes, as if nodding 'yes' (sagittal plane), shaking 'no' (horizontal plane) & head bobbing side to side, ear-to-shoulder and back (frontal plane), aka 'the Indian head-shake'.

Repetitions: 3 – 5

Tip: Move slowly

Ignore any sounds from neck so long as they are painless

Stop and skip if uncomfortable or hurting.

Your shoulders would tend to shrug up at the last movement, but your arms interlocked behind your back would ensure they remain low and relaxed.

3D-HEAD ROLLS & SHAKES
शिरग्रीवासंचालनम्

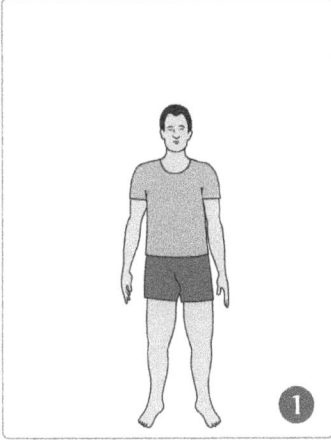

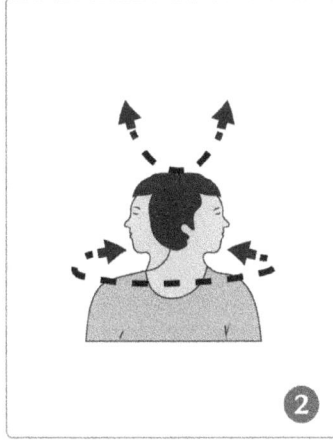

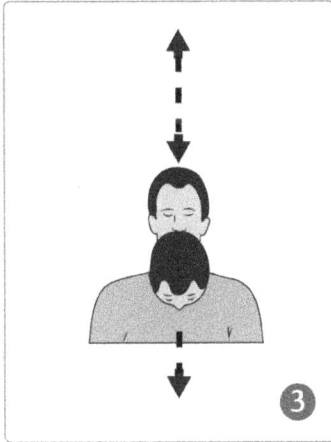

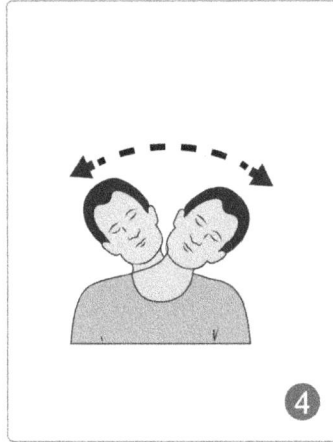

7

DETAILED DESCRIPTION OF EACH ACTIVITY: PART 2 (OTHER POSTURES)

"I need to be fit to feel easy"
— Jurgen Klinsmann, Footballer

"An 'Iron will' is always supported by fitness"
— Ivan Lendl, Tennis star

Detailed description of each activity: Part 2 (Other postures, etc.)

On the fours: palms & knees:

13 3D-head shakes:

Body posture:	crawling on all fours, resting on two palms and two knees
Head:	facing the floor, looking ahead at the floor,
Arms:	straight at elbows,
Knees:	bent at right angle, toes touching the floor
Activity:	Shake your head along three axes, as if nodding 'yes' (sagittal plane), shaking 'no' (frontal plane) & head bobbing side to side, ear-to-shoulder and back, (horizontal plane).
Repetitions:	3 – 5
Tip:	Move slowly.
	Ignore any sounds from neck so long as they are painless.
	Stop and skip if uncomfortable or hurting.
	You may feel the movement in the muscles by the side of your spine and your back relaxing.

3D-HEAD ROTATION IN CRAWLING
शिरग्रीवासंचालनम्

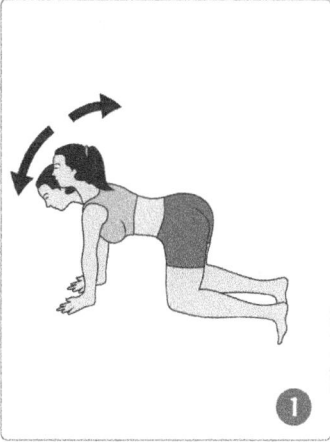

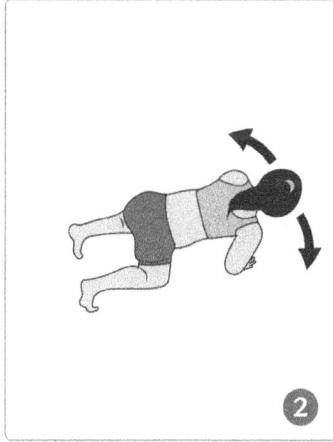

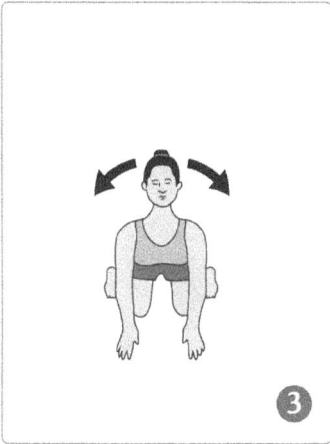

14 Sole claps:

Body posture:	crawling on all fours, resting on two palms and two knees
Head:	facing the floor, looking ahead at the floor
Arms:	straight at elbows,
Knees:	bent at right angle, toes touching the floor.
Activity:	Lift your feet off the floor and pivoting on the knees, clap your soles, cupping them alternately.
Repetitions:	5 – 15
Tip:	Ensure good padding under your knees for best comfort.

SOLE CLAPS:
पदतालिका

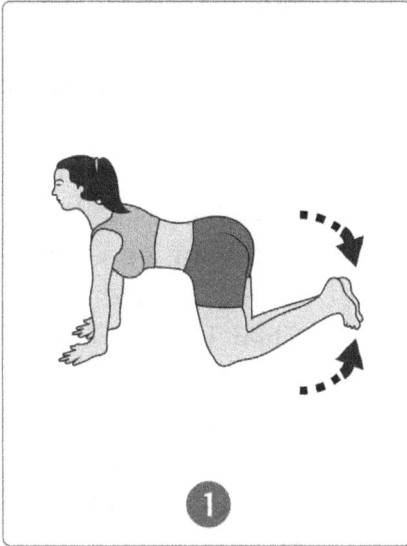

15 Pony-kicks:

Body posture:	crawling on all fours, resting on two palms and two knees
Head:	lifted, looking ahead in front
Arms:	straight at elbows,
Knees:	bent at right angle, toes touching the floor.
Activity:	Lift one knee bending it up to your chest & kick back forcefully as if your leg is a javelin missile to be launched at the back.
	Then kick back with the other knee.
Repetitions:	5 – 10 continuously.
Tip:	Ensure good padding under your knees for best comfort.
	Your hip should tilt slightly to the opposite side to give ground-clearance to your knee as it passes closest to the floor.

PONY-KICKS
अश्वलत्ता - वक्षजानुप्रक्षेपणम्

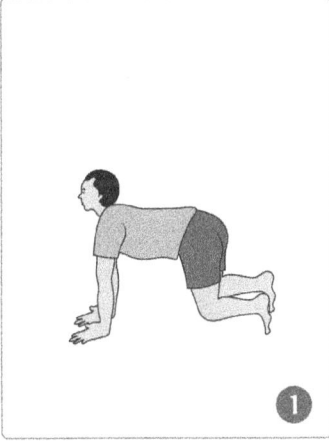

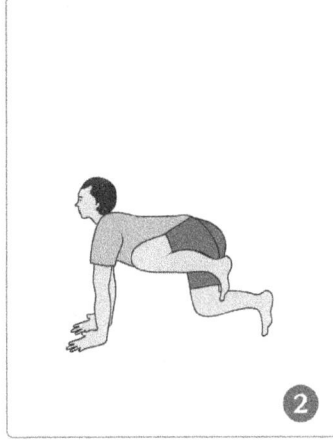

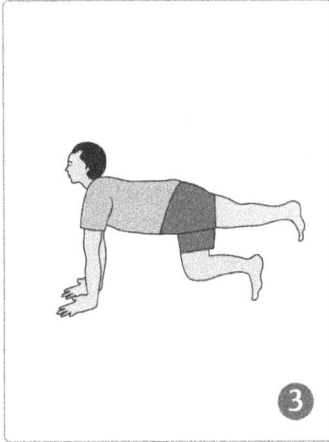

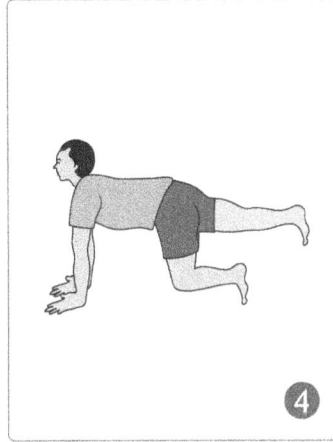

16 Push ups:

Body posture:	crawling on all fours, resting on two palms and two soles.
Head:	facing the floor, looking ahead at the floor
Arms:	straight at elbows,
Knees:	straight, soles touching the floor.
Activity:	**'Standard push-up':** Gently exhale while lowering your face towards the floor by bending the elbows until your nose barely touches the floor, then straighten the elbows while inhaling, to revert to starting posture.
Repetitions:	5 – 15
Tip:	Start slowly, even with one push up and increase slowly by one extra push up every week.
	Your lowering and lifting movement of head and shoulders would draw or describe a circle.

PUSH UPS
जोर - भुजाशीर्षोत्थापनम्

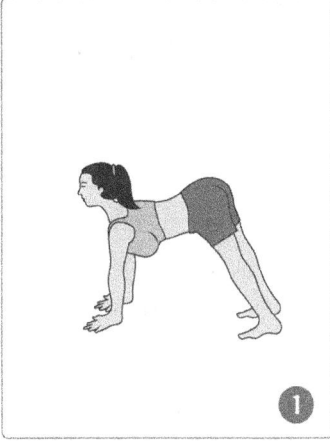

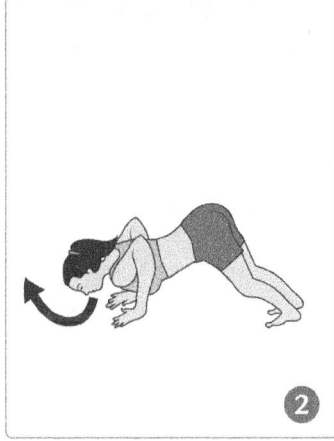

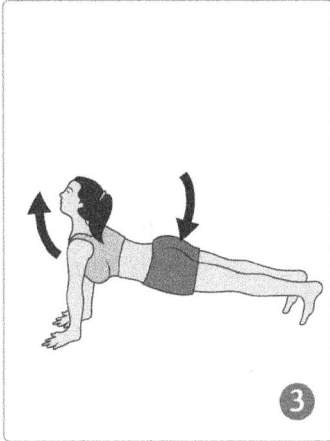

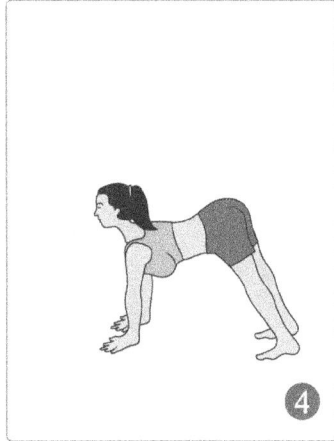

Supine: on a firm flat surface, thin mat or rug:

17   Raised leg movements: Toe-curling

Body posture:	flat on your back
Head:	rested, looking ahead at the ceiling or sky
Arms:	by the side, straight at elbows
Knees:	straight
Activity:	Raise both legs off the floor from hips with straight knees and draw circles & a figure- eight with toes clockwise and then anticlockwise.
	Total four types of movements.
Repetitions:	3 – 7 continuously x4
Tip:	You may find this rather tough at the beginning.
	You should see your toes just in the periphery of your visual field looking straight ahead, to ensure the circles are big enough and helpful.
	When you can do all the circles and figure eights in one go without touching the floor, you have crunched it!

TOE-CURLING
पादचक्रम्

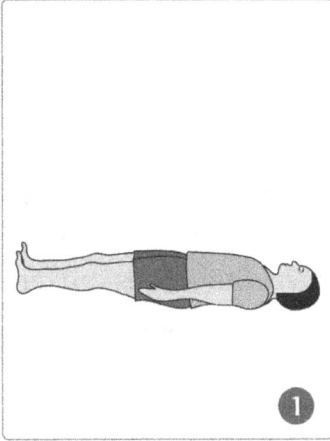

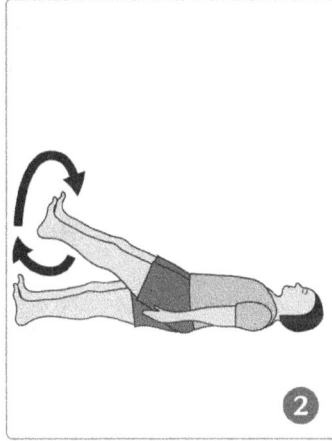

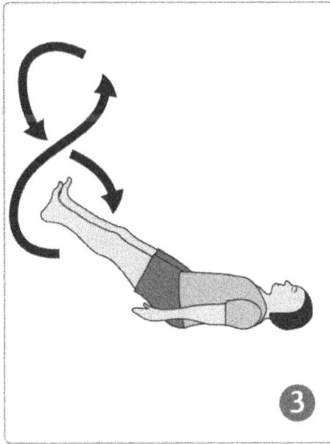

18 **Knee-diamond butterfly**:

Body posture: flat on your back.

Head: rested, looking ahead at the ceiling or sky.

Arms: by the side, straight at elbows.

Knees: bent, so as both soles can touch each other.

Activity: Join the soles together to make a diamond of your thighs and legs. Then move the knees up and down off the ground, without banging them on the floor.

Repetitions: 5 – 10 continuously.

KNEE-DIAMOND BUTTERFLY
पदतलचुंबित जानुचक्रम्

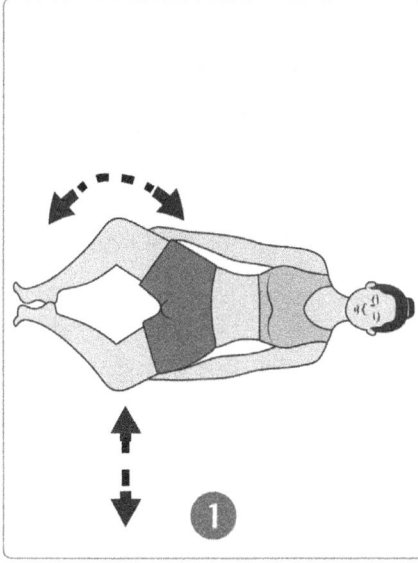

19 **Bundled up**:

Body posture	flat on your back.
Head:	rested, looking ahead at the ceiling or sky.
Arms:	in front, fingers firmly interlocked.
Knees:	bent, so as both soles can touch each other.
Activity:	Join the soles together to make a diamond of your thighs and legs. Then lift the joined soles towards your face and grab them in your clasped interlocked palms.
Repetitions:	Hold this position for x3 deep slow breaths.
Tip:	You may rock your head off the floor in this posture 3-5 times and feel your upper spine relaxing and 'resetting'.

BUNDLED UP
पदावगुंठित पवनमुक्तासन

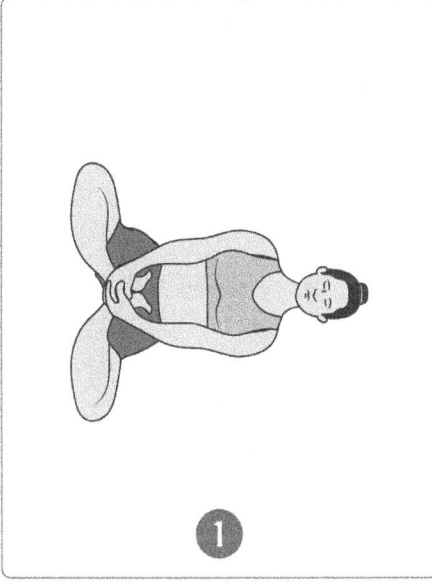

20 DIY-back massage:

Body posture: flat on your back.

Head: rested, looking ahead at the ceiling or sky.

Arms: in front, fingers firmly interlocked.

Knees: bent, so as both soles can touch each other.

Activity: While 'bundled up' as in **#19** above (Join the soles together to make a diamond of your thighs and legs, lift the joined soles towards your face and grab them in your clasped interlocked palms), roll side-by-side until thighs touch the floor on one side and then you roll back to the opposite side, rocking gently and continuously.

Repetitions: 5 – 10+ continuously, as many as you like!

Tip: You may feel your back muscles gently squeezed between your ribcage and the floor.

DIY-BACK MASSAGE
पदावगुंठित स्वपृष्ठमर्दनम्

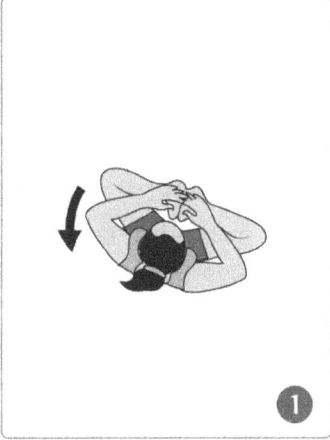

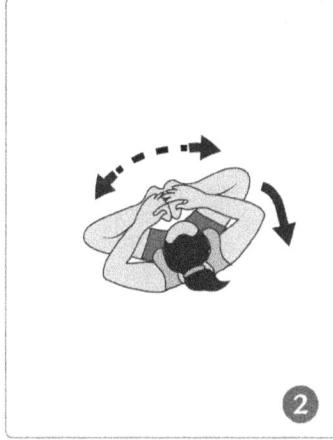

21 Winding down: Relax!

Body posture: flat on your back.

Head: rested, eyes closed.

Arms: by the side, straight at elbows.

Knees: straight, heels touching the floor.

Activity: None. Just RELAX! Imagine yourself as a feather, a butterfly, a sycamore seed whirling weightlessly in the breeze; recall & re-live the best moments from yesterday…

Repetitions: x3 deep slow breaths or more.

Tip: You may feel more relaxed with varying, colourful, musical memory routines.

WINDING DOWN: RELAXATION
विश्राम

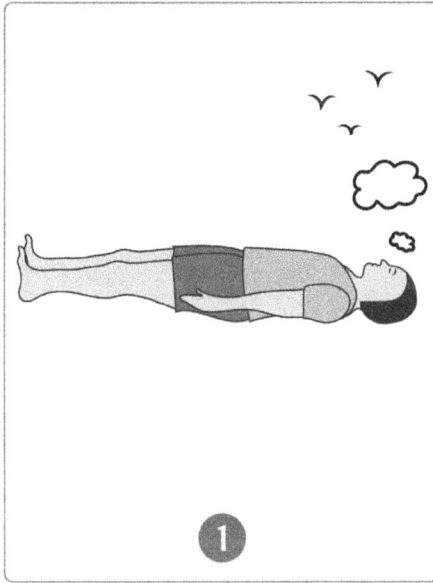

Standing up again ('getting ready for the day!')

22 **Sit ups**:

Body posture:	standing, feet wider apart, pointing outwards.
Head:	facing forward, looking ahead.
Arms:	by the side,
Palms:	facing the body or in soft fists.
Activity:	Holding opposite ear-lobules in your index finger & thumb, that is elbows crossed in front, squat down on the floor with bending knees fully and get up.
Repetitions:	10 – 25 continuous.
Tip:	Start slowly, with 3 or 5 sit-ups at the beginning and increase slowly by two extra sit ups every week.

SIT-UPS
उपविशोत्तिष्ठकम्

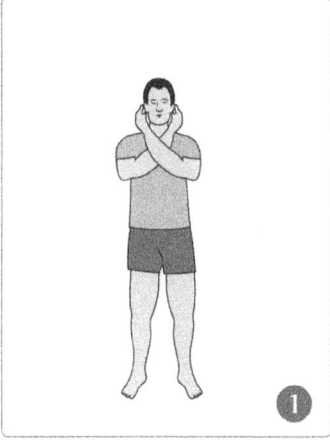

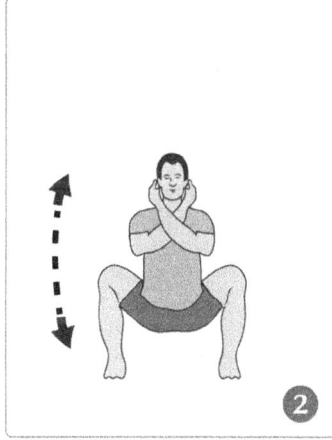

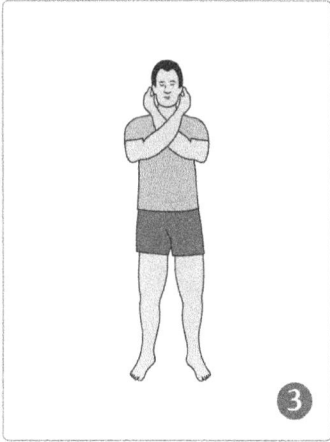

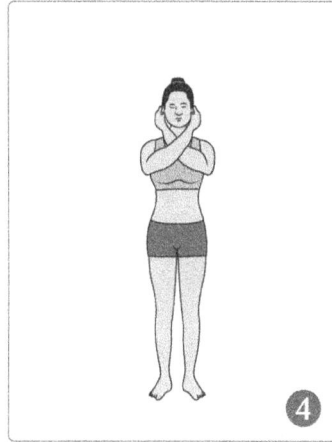

23 Backward arm rotations:

Body posture: standing, feet shoulder-width apart.

Head: facing forward, looking ahead.

Arms: by the side.

Palms: facing the body, or rolled in soft fists.

Activity: Swing both arms forwards, raise overhead and down from the back, to draw full circle in the air with your hands or fists.

Repetitions: 10 – 20 continuous, non-stop.

Tip: This action is exactly opposite of **#6.**

BACKWARD ARM-SWINGS
अवस्कंधचक्रम्

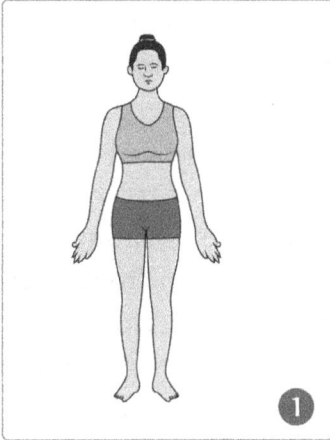

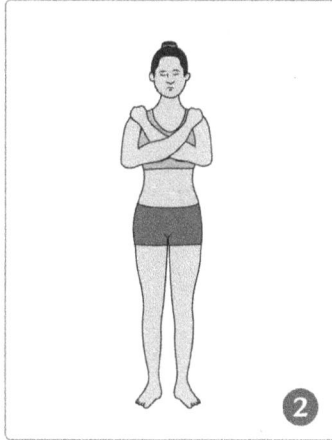

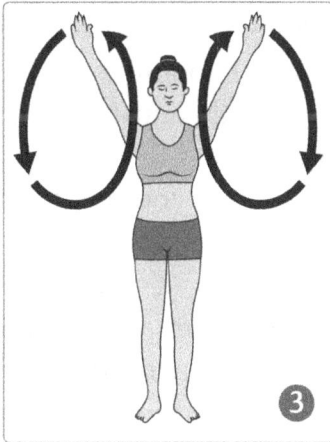

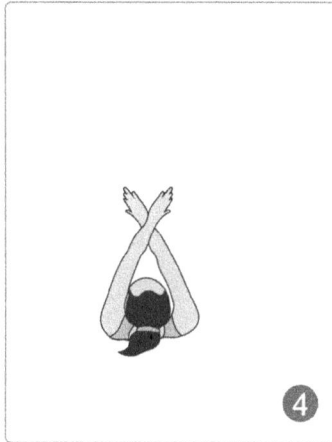

24 SRT: Sitting-rising test:

Body posture: standing, feet shoulder-width apart.

Head: facing forward, looking ahead.

Arms: elbows crossed in front, pinching opposite ear-lobules.

Legs: crossed like scissors.

Activity: Holding opposite ear-lobules in your index finger & thumb, that is elbows crossed in front, squat down on the floor cross-legged without losing your footing and bending knees fully. Now get up by reversing this movement and without losing your balance.

Repetitions: Once-a-day is enough!

Tip: This is trickier than just walking on a straight line.

You 'pass' even if you squat and get up.

Super-advanced, if you can 'ground' your bum and get up! This test is used by neurologists to quickly assess posture, strength, balance and coordination all in one go.

SITTING-RISING TEST
संकरितोपविशोत्तिष्ठकम्

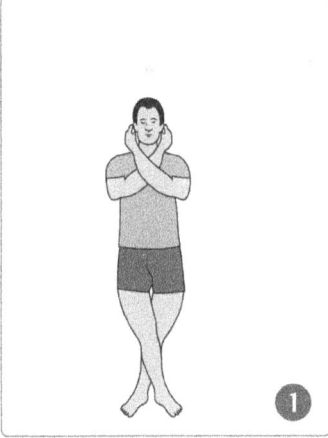

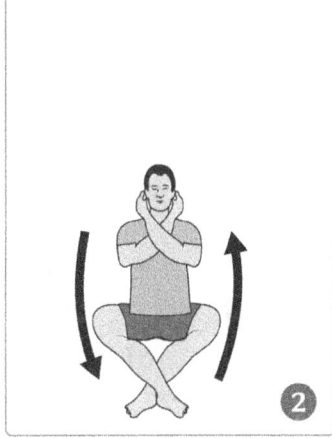

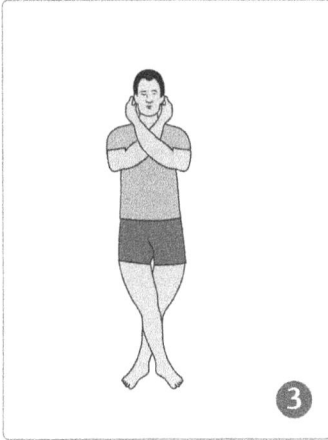

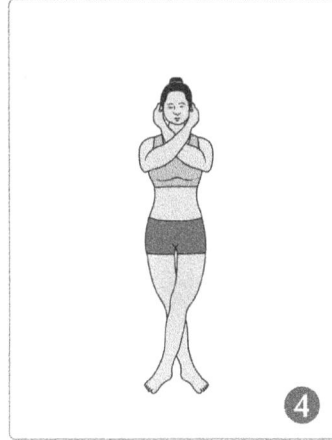

25 SUOOL: Standing up on one leg:

Body posture: sitting on a chair or bench.

Head: facing forward, looking ahead.

Arms: folded, elbows crossed in front.

Legs: neutral, feet bent at the knees.

Activity: Raising one leg off the ground straight in front of you, try & get up and stand on the other leg, without using arms or losing your balance.

Repetitions: Once on either foot.

Tip: This is impossible to do if your perch is short and knee bent less than 90 degrees.

Move your standing foot slightly under the seat of chair or bench to maintain gravity.

Stretch the non-standing leg as far straight to gain balance.

Try putting your raised leg across opposite knee or thigh.

This test is also used by neurologists to quickly assess posture, strength, balance and coordination all in one go.

STANDING UP ON EITHER LEG
एकपादोत्तिष्ठकम्

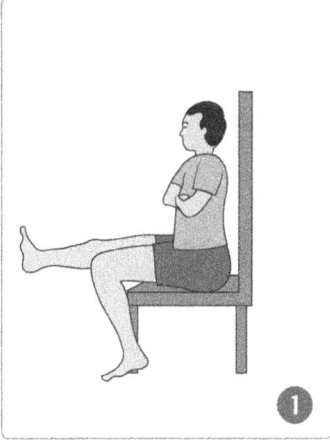

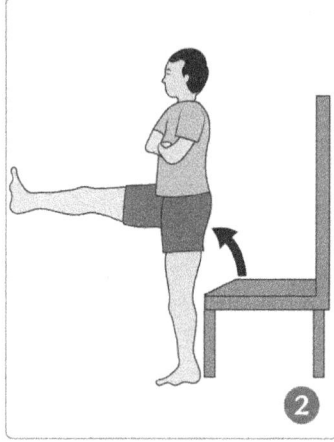

8

SANSKRIT NAMES FOR GYMLESS FITNESS ACTIVITIES

"Fitness is not about being better than someone else. It's about being better than YOU used to be."
"The secret of getting ahead is getting started."
— Mark Twain

Sanskrit names & Deonagari spellings for Gymless Fitness activities:

Standing (biped): Dwipadawastha – द्वपिादावस्था , उत्तष्ठिावस्था

1. Sky-scratch: Tadasan - ताडासन

2. Selfie-commend: Aparhastprushthasparsham - अपरहस्तपृष्ठस्पर्शम्

3. Sun-salutes – sooryanamaskar - सूर्यनमस्कार
   (include:
   Frog pose: Mandookawastha - मंडूकावस्था,
   Cobra poise – Bhujangawastha - भुजंगावस्था,
   One-knee-bent posture –
   Ekajanuwakshapranipat – एकजानुवक्षपरणिपात:

4. Elbow thrusts-by-side: Ardhagomukham - अर्धगोमुखम्

5. Straight arm-swings-by-twist: Katichakram - कटिचक्रम्

6. Forward arm rotations: Skandhachakram - स्कंधचक्रम्
   Includes: Cupping opposite shoulders:
   Aparaskandhasparsham - अपरस्कन्धस्पर्शम्

7. Spider-web spin: Tantunabhika - तंतुनाभिका

8. Elephant trunk & head shakes:
   Hastishundashirandolanam - हस्तिशुंडाशिरांदोलनम्

9. Butterfly-thrusts: Prajapati-shalabhika - प्रजापति शलभिका

10. Dragonfly-thrusts: Vyadhapatangakam - व्याधपतंगकम्

11. Sky-mining / Cheetah sprint:
    Upavyaghraratham - उपव्याघ्ररथम्

12. 3D-head rolls & shakes:
    Shiragreewasanchalanam - शिरिग्रीवासंचालनम्
    On all fours (palms and knees, Quadruped):
    Chatushpadawastha - चतुष्पादावस्था

13. 3D-head shakes: Greewasanchalanam - ग्रीवासंचालनम्

14. Sole claps: Padatalika – पदतालिका

15. Pony-kicks: Ashwalatta – अश्वलत्तता

16. Wakshajanuprakshepanam - वक्षजानुप्रक्षेपणम्

17. Push ups: Jor - जोर – Bhujasheershotthaapanam
    - भुजाशीर्षोत्थापनम्

18. Toe-curling: Padachakre - पादचक्रम्,

19. Knee-diamond butterfly: Padatalachumbit
    januchakram - पदतलचुंबति जानुचक्रम्

20. Bundled up: Padawagunthit pawanamuktasan -
    पदावगुंठति पवनमुक्तासन

21. DIY-back massage: Padawagunthit
    swaprushthamardanam - पदावगुंठति
    स्वपृष्ठमर्दनम्

22. Winding down relaxation: Wishwam - विश्राम:

23. Sit-ups: Baithak – बैठक, Upawishottishthakam -
    उपवशिोत्तषि्ठकम्

24. Backward arm-swings: Awaskandhachakram -
    अवस्कंधचक्रम्

25. Sitting-Rising Test :
    Sangkaritopawishottishthakam -
    सङ्करतिोपवशिोत्तषि्ठकम्

26. Standing up from sitting on one leg:
    Ekapadottishthakam - एकपादोत्तषि्ठकम्

9

NO TIME FOR GYM?
GET THE VIDEOS!

"Get off your COVID-Coma-Couch & work with me"
                – Loral Langermeier Millionaire Maker &
                            one of stars of 'The Secret'

*"TV can make you rich or poor. Poor when it's ON,
rich when it's OFF!"*

Congratulations, reader, for knowing of *Gymless Fitness.*

Some of us think with the right side of the brain and understand visual instruction better. Of course, the diagrams speak 1000 words, but the videos of the activities performed by untrained everyday persons as well as the author speak a million words.

Why not grab the videos?

A custom made set of 3 concise
videos is available for **$99** at:
TheGymlessFitness.com

As a thank you for purchasing the book, use the discount code at the below link and access the videos at less than half price!

Only **$49**.

Yogolution.com

Link to YouTube introductory video:

https://youtu.be/6fCZ5w9hAlw

10

SPREAD THE MESSAGE – LIVE IN A FITTER WORLD!

"I need to be fit to feel easy"
　　　　　　　　　　– Jurgen Klinsmann, Footballer

"An 'Iron will' is always supported by fitness"
　　　　　　　　　　　　– Ivan Lendl, Tennis star

And finally, how would you like to benefit from this book in addition to getting and remaining fit?

For information on how to share the knowledge and information in this book for the benefit of others, please visit:
TheGymlessFitness.com

Check out our affiliate program, group coaching, and premium level one-to-one coaching.

Here is to a fitter, healthier, happier and prosperous future.

Chapter 11

BORING BUT ESSENTIAL (DISCLAIMERS)

"Exercise is done against one's wishes and maintained only because the alternative is worse."
– George A Sheehan

"Motivation is the art of getting people to do what you want them to do because they want to do it."
– Dwight Eisenhower

Here's the boring but essential: Statutory Disclaimers:

1. Although I am a doctor: trained physician, the information I provide here is specific to Gymless Fitness activities and is based on my personal experience, studies of anatomy & physiology and my experience of actually performing these over the past twenty years.

2. The information contained in our website, blog, guest blogs, e-mails, programs, services and/ or products like this video is for educational and informational purposes only, and is made available to you as self-help tools for your own use. While we draw on our prior professional expertise and background in many areas, you

acknowledge that we are supporting you in our roles exclusively as remote exercise coaches only. We provide information concerning, but not limited to Gymless Fitness through 21st century Evol-Yoga.

3. We aim to accurately represent the information provided on this website, blog, e-mails, programs, services, and products. You are acknowledging that you are participating voluntarily in using our website or blog or in any of our e-mails, programs, services, and/or products, and you alone are solely and personally responsible for your results. You acknowledge that you take full responsibility for your health, life and well-being, as well as the health, lives and well-being of your family and children (born and unborn, as applicable), and all decisions now or in the future.

4. In the event that you use the information provided through our website, blog, e-mails, programs, services, and/or products, we assume no responsibility or liability of any nature.

5. Every effort is made to ensure the accuracy of published information on or through our website, blog, e-mails, programs, services and products; however, any unintended errors are regretted and excepted. We shall always endeavour to present you with the most accurate, up-to-date information, but we cannot be held responsible for the accuracy of the content that is constantly evolving due to research in this field.

Particularly, I, Dr Shree, am not in a position to diagnose your symptoms or provide you medical advice except by private consultation, which is NOT part of Gymless Fitness Activities.

RESULTS DISCLAIMERS

1. We make every effort to ensure that we accurately represent these products and services and their potential for results. There is no guarantee that you will experience the same results and you accept the risk that fitness results may differ by individual. We make no guarantees concerning the level of success you may achieve, and you accept the risk that results will differ for each individual.

2. Each individual's health, fitness, and nutrition success depends on his or her background, motivation, commitment and regularity.

3. The use of our information, products and services should be based on your own due diligence and you agree that our company is not liable for any success or failure of your physique that is directly or indirectly related to the purchase and use of our information, products and services.

4. We present real world experiences and insights on other people's experiences for purposes of illustration only.

5. The testimonials, examples, and photos used are of actual clients and results they personally achieved. Each client has approved these

testimonials, examples, and photos for use in materials to speak to our program, service, and/or product capabilities, but they are not intended to represent or guarantee that current or future clients will achieve the same results. Rather, these client stories represent what is possible with our programs, services, and/or products.

Links, et cetera.

As stated in the website and in addition, we are not responsible for the contents of any off-site webpages, companies or persons linked or referenced in this site. Reference or links in the website, blog, e-mails, programs, services or products to any other business or entity's information, opinions, advice, programs, services, or products do not constitute our endorsement or recommendation.

www.ingramcontent.com/pod-product-compliance
Lightning Source LLC
Chambersburg PA
CBHW070126030426
42335CB00016B/2284